Table of Contents

Introduction

Welcome to "Home Gym Fitness Blueprint: The Smart Setup for Success"! I'm excited to be your guide as we embark on this journey to create a home gym that will help you achieve your fitness goals. Whether you're a beginner looking to establish a fitness routine or an experienced gym-goer seeking the convenience of working out at home, this book is designed to provide you with the knowledge and inspiration you need to build a personalized home gym setup.

Why a Home Gym?

In today's fast-paced world, finding the time and motivation to go to a traditional gym can be challenging. With a home gym, you have the convenience of working out whenever you want, without the hassle of travel time or membership fees. A well-designed home gym can save you money in the long run, as you won't need to pay for monthly gym memberships or expensive fitness classes. Plus, having your own space means you can tailor it to your specific needs and preferences, making your workouts more enjoyable and effective.

What This Book Covers

We'll start by helping you define your fitness goals and assess your available space and budget. It's important to have a clear understanding of what you want to achieve and the resources you have before you start setting up your home gym. We'll guide you through the process of selecting essential equipment, optimizing your space and layout for maximum efficiency, and making the most of what you have.

Next, we'll delve into creating effective workout routines that target various muscle groups and cater to your specific fitness goals. We'll explore the concept of progressive overload, which is crucial for continuous growth and improvement, and show you how to incorporate cardiovascular training to enhance your overall fitness.

Flexibility and mobility are essential components of any fitness routine, so we'll dedicate a chapter to focusing on these aspects. We'll provide you with stretching and mobility exercises that will help prevent injuries and improve your overall athletic performance.

Establishing a routine and maintaining consistency is vital for long-term success in any fitness journey. We'll guide you through the process of establishing a workout routine that suits your lifestyle and preferences. We'll also discuss how to evolve your home gym setup as your fitness level and goals change over time.

How to Use This Book

Throughout this book, you'll find practical tips, expert advice, and inspirational stories to keep you motivated and engaged in your fitness journey. We encourage you to take ownership of your health and well-being by creating a home gym that is tailored to your needs and preferences.

Defining Your Fitness Goals

Before you start buying equipment and rearranging your space, take some time to think about what you want to achieve with your home gym. Are you looking to build muscle, lose weight, improve your cardiovascular health, or increase flexibility? Your goals will help determine the type of equipment you need and the best way to set up your space.

Assessing Your Space and Budget

Next, assess the space you have available for your home gym. Do you have a dedicated room, or will you be setting up in a corner of your living room or garage? Consider the size of the space and how much equipment you can realistically fit. Also, think about your budget. How much are you willing to spend on your home gym setup? Remember, you don't need to buy everything at once. You can start with a few essential pieces and add more over time as your budget allows.

Selecting Essential Equipment

Once you have a clear understanding of your goals, space, and budget, it's time to select your equipment. We'll guide you through choosing the essential items that will help you achieve your fitness goals. From resistance bands and dumbbells to stability balls and cardio machines, we'll cover all the basics and explain how each piece of equipment can be used effectively.

Optimizing Your Space

Creating an efficient and organized workout space is key to making the most of your home gym. We'll provide tips on how to arrange your equipment, store your gear, and create a motivating environment. A well-organized space will make your workouts more enjoyable and help you stay consistent.

Building Effective Workout Routines

With your equipment in place, we'll show you how to create workout routines that target different muscle groups and align with your fitness goals. We'll explore the concept of progressive overload, which involves gradually increasing the intensity of your workouts to continue making progress. Additionally, we'll cover how to incorporate cardiovascular training into your routines to boost your overall fitness.

Flexibility and Mobility Exercises

To prevent injuries and improve your athletic performance, it's essential to include flexibility and mobility exercises in your routine. We'll provide a variety of stretching and mobility exercises that you can incorporate into your workouts to keep your body flexible and resilient.

Establishing a Routine and Maintaining Consistency

Consistency is key to achieving your fitness goals. We'll guide you through the process of establishing a workout routine that fits your lifestyle and preferences. Whether you prefer morning workouts or evening sessions, we'll help you create a schedule that you can stick to.

Evolving Your Home Gym Setup

As your fitness level and goals evolve, so should your home gym setup. We'll discuss how to adapt your space and equipment to meet your changing needs. Whether you want to add new equipment, rearrange your space, or try new workout routines, we'll provide tips and inspiration to keep your home gym fresh and effective.

Conclusion

Building a home gym is an investment in your health and well-being. By creating a space that is tailored to your needs and preferences, you can enjoy the convenience and flexibility of working out at home. This book will provide you with the knowledge and inspiration you need to create a successful home gym setup and achieve your fitness goals. So, let's dive in and start building your dream home gym!

Chapter 1: Defining Your Fitness Goals

Before you embark on creating an effective and successful home gym setup, it's essential to start by defining your fitness goals. By clearly identifying what you want to achieve through your workouts, you will be able to tailor your equipment selection, workout routines, and overall approach to meet those specific objectives.

Understanding the Importance of Setting Goals

Setting goals is crucial because it provides you with direction and motivation. When you have a clear purpose in mind, it becomes easier to stay focused and committed to your fitness journey. Whether your aim is to lose weight, build muscle, improve cardiovascular endurance, enhance flexibility, or simply maintain overall fitness, having well-defined goals will greatly increase your chances of success.

In this chapter, we will explore the key steps to effectively define your fitness goals:

1. Reflect on Your Personal Aspirations

Take some time to think about what you truly want to achieve with your fitness routine. Consider both short-term and long-term goals. Are you looking to improve your physical appearance, boost your energy levels, or enhance your athletic performance? Understanding your personal aspirations will help you align your efforts with what truly matters to you.

Ask yourself questions like:

- Do I want to lose a specific amount of weight?
- Am I aiming to build muscle or tone my body?
- Is my primary focus on improving my cardiovascular health?
- Do I want to increase my flexibility or balance?
- Am I preparing for a specific event or sport?

2. Set SMART Goals

SMART stands for Specific, Measurable, Attainable, Relevant, and Time-bound. When setting your fitness goals, make sure they meet these criteria. For example, instead of saying "I want to get stronger," a SMART goal would be "I want to increase my bench press by 10 pounds within the next 3 months." This gives you a specific target to aim for and a clear timeline to track your progress.

- **Specific:** Clearly define what you want to accomplish.

- **Measurable:** Ensure you can track your progress and know when you've achieved your goal.
- **Attainable:** Set realistic goals that are challenging yet achievable.
- **Relevant:** Choose goals that are meaningful and align with your overall objectives.
- **Time-bound:** Set a deadline to create a sense of urgency and motivation.

3. Prioritize Your Goals

If you have multiple fitness goals, it's important to prioritize them based on their significance to you. This will help you allocate your time and resources effectively. For instance, if weight loss is your primary goal, you may need to focus more on cardiovascular exercises and adjust your nutrition accordingly.

Consider which goals will have the most impact on your health and happiness and prioritize them. This approach ensures that you make consistent progress in the areas that matter most to you.

4. Write Down Your Goals

Studies have shown that writing down your goals increases the likelihood of achieving them. By putting your goals on paper, you make them tangible and create a sense of commitment. Keep your written goals somewhere visible, such as on your refrigerator or near your home gym area, to serve as a daily reminder of what you're working towards.

Writing down your goals not only solidifies your commitment but also helps you stay focused and motivated. It becomes a constant visual cue to keep you on track.

5. Be Realistic and Flexible

While it's important to challenge yourself, it's also crucial to be realistic about what you can achieve. Set goals that are attainable and consider your current fitness level, time availability, and any potential limitations or constraints. Additionally, be open to adjusting your goals as you progress and evolve in your fitness journey.

Flexibility in your goals allows you to adapt to changes in your life, such as a new work schedule, family commitments, or unexpected challenges. This adaptability ensures that you continue to make progress without becoming discouraged.

Conclusion

By following these steps, you will establish clear and meaningful fitness goals that will guide your entire home gym setup. Having a strong sense of purpose will not only keep you motivated but also ensure that you design a setup that aligns perfectly with your aspirations. Defining your fitness goals is the foundation upon which you will build your fitness journey.

Continue reading to discover how to assess your space and budget for your home gym setup in Chapter 2.

Chapter 2: Assessing Your Space and Budget

When creating a home gym, it's essential to assess your available space and budget. By carefully evaluating these factors, you can ensure that you optimize your fitness setup and make wise decisions regarding equipment and layout.

Evaluating Your Space

Start by measuring the space you have allocated for your home gym. Take note of the dimensions and any potential obstacles or limitations, such as low ceilings or uneven floors. This information will help you determine what type and size of equipment will fit comfortably in your space.

Consider the layout and flow of the room. It's important to have enough space to move around freely and perform exercises without feeling cramped. Additionally, ensure there is ample ventilation and lighting for a pleasant and comfortable workout environment. Good lighting can make a big difference in your motivation and energy levels during workouts.

Think about the different zones you might need within your gym space. For example, you might want a dedicated area for cardio equipment, another for weight training, and a separate space for stretching or yoga. This can help you visualize how to arrange your equipment and maintain an efficient flow in your workout routines.

Assessing Your Budget

Determining your budget is another crucial aspect of setting up a home gym. Consider how much you are willing and able to invest in your fitness regimen. Setting a budget will help guide your purchasing decisions and prevent overspending.

Remember to consider not only the upfront costs but also the long-term expenses. This may include equipment maintenance, replacement parts, and any necessary accessories or upgrades. It's essential to factor in these costs to ensure the sustainability of your home gym.

Think about your fitness priorities and allocate your budget accordingly. For example, if strength training is your primary focus, investing in a good set of adjustable dumbbells or a quality weight bench might be a top priority. If you enjoy cardio workouts, a treadmill or stationary bike could be a worthwhile investment.

Maximizing Your Space and Budget

Once you have assessed your space and budget, it's time to optimize them for maximum effectiveness. Here are some strategies to make the most of both:

Prioritize Essential Equipment

Identify the key pieces of equipment that align with your fitness goals. Focus on investing in high-quality items that provide versatile workout options. For example, a set of resistance bands can be used for a variety of exercises targeting different muscle groups, making them a valuable addition to any home gym.

Consider Multifunctional Equipment

Look for equipment that serves multiple purposes. Adjustable dumbbells, for instance, can replace an entire rack of individual weights, saving both space and money. Resistance bands and kettlebells are also versatile tools that can be used in numerous ways to enhance your workouts.

Explore Space-Saving Options

If you have limited space, consider compact or foldable equipment that can be easily stored when not in use. Wall-mounted racks or storage systems can help keep your gym area organized and maximize floor space. Items like foldable treadmills or collapsible weight benches are excellent choices for small spaces.

Shop for Deals and Discounts

Keep an eye out for sales, promotions, and second-hand options. Many fitness equipment retailers offer discounts throughout the year, allowing you to snag excellent deals on quality equipment. Websites like Craigslist, Facebook Marketplace, or dedicated fitness forums often have gently used equipment at a fraction of the cost of new items.

DIY Solutions

Get creative with DIY solutions to save money. For example, you can use household items like water jugs or backpacks filled with books as makeshift weights. Building your own plyometric box or squat rack with basic materials can also be a cost-effective way to enhance your home gym without breaking the bank.

Conclusion

By carefully assessing your space and budget, you can make informed decisions about the equipment and layout of your home gym. This will help you create an effective and efficient fitness environment that aligns with your goals without breaking the bank.

Remember, a home gym doesn't need to be extravagant to be effective. Focus on your fitness priorities, invest in quality equipment, and make the most of the space you have. In the next chapter, we'll delve into specific equipment recommendations and layout ideas to help you get started on building your ideal home gym.

Chapter 3: Selecting Essential Equipment

When it comes to setting up your home gym, selecting the right equipment is crucial. The right tools can make or break your fitness journey. In this chapter, we'll explore the essential equipment you need to set up a functional and effective home gym.

Understanding Your Fitness Goals

Before diving into the world of home gym equipment, it's important to understand your fitness goals. Are you looking to build strength, improve cardiovascular fitness, or focus on flexibility? Different goals require different equipment, so it's essential to identify what you want to achieve before making any purchases.

Strength Training Equipment

Strength training is a vital component of any fitness routine. To effectively target different muscle groups, consider investing in a set of dumbbells or adjustable weights. These versatile tools allow you to adjust the resistance and cater to your strength level.

- **Dumbbells or Adjustable Weights:** These are versatile tools that allow you to adjust the resistance and cater to your strength level. They are perfect for a variety of exercises that target different muscle groups.

- **Weight Bench:** A weight bench is another essential piece of equipment for strength training. It provides a stable surface for exercises such as bench presses, step-ups, and tricep dips. Look for a bench that can be adjusted to different incline levels to add variety to your workouts.
- **Power Rack or Squat Rack:** If you have the space and budget, a power rack or squat rack is an excellent addition to your home gym. It allows you to perform compound exercises such as squats, bench presses, and pull-ups safely and effectively.

Cardiovascular Equipment

Cardiovascular exercises are essential for improving your heart health and burning calories. There are various options for incorporating cardiovascular equipment into your home gym.

- **Treadmills, Ellipticals, and Stationary Bikes:** These machines provide excellent cardio workouts. Consider your space limitations and personal preferences when choosing the right equipment for you.
- **Jump Ropes and Mini Trampolines:** If space is a concern, jump ropes and mini trampolines are excellent alternatives for

cardiovascular exercises. They are
compact, portable, and can provide an
effective and intense workout.

Functional Training Equipment

Functional training focuses on improving your
overall body movements and strength for everyday
activities. Here are some essential tools for
functional training:

- **Resistance Bands:** These are great for
  improving strength and flexibility. They are
  also very portable and easy to store.
- **Stability Balls and Medicine Balls:** These
  tools help improve balance, stability, and
  core strength.
- **Suspension Trainers (e.g., TRX Straps):**
  These are versatile and can be attached to
  doors, walls, or ceiling mounts. They allow
  you to perform a wide variety of exercises
  using your body weight.

Additional Considerations

When selecting equipment for your home gym,
remember to consider the quality and durability of
the products. Investing in high-quality equipment
will ensure longevity and prevent the need for
frequent replacements.

- **Quality and Durability:** Investing in high-quality equipment ensures longevity and prevents the need for frequent replacements.
- **Skill Level and Long-term Goals:** As you progress in your fitness journey, you may need to upgrade or add new equipment to challenge yourself further. Plan for future expansion and make room for growth in your home gym setup.
- **Safety:** Don't forget about safety. Make sure to have proper flooring, such as rubber mats or interlocking foam tiles, to reduce the risk of injury and protect your equipment.

Conclusion

Choosing the right equipment for your home gym is a critical step in setting yourself up for success. By understanding your fitness goals, prioritizing essential equipment, and considering versatility and durability, you can create a well-rounded and functional home gym. In the next chapter, we'll dive into optimizing space and layout to ensure you make the most of your home gym setup.

Chapter 4: Optimizing Space and Layout

Hey there! Setting up a home gym can be a game-changer for your fitness routine, but one of the most critical aspects is optimizing the space and layout. A well-organized and efficient space not only enhances your workout experience but also ensures you have enough room to perform exercises safely and effectively. Let's dive into the details and make the most out of your home gym space.

Measuring Your Space

Before you start rearranging furniture and purchasing equipment, it's crucial to measure the available space in your designated area. Grab a tape measure and take precise measurements of the room dimensions, including length, width, and height. Don't forget to note any limitations like low ceilings, narrow doorways, or limited floor space. Having these measurements handy will help you plan better and avoid any surprises later on.

Considering Layout

With your measurements in hand, it's time to think about the layout of your home gym. Visualize the flow of movement and how various equipment pieces will fit together. You want to ensure there's enough room to move freely and perform exercises without feeling cramped. Think about how you'll transition between different exercises and whether the layout supports a smooth flow.

Dividing the Space

Dividing the space into different zones can help create a well-organized and functional layout. Consider designating specific areas for different types of workouts, such as:

- **Cardio Equipment Zone**: Place treadmills, stationary bikes, or rowing machines here.
- **Strength Training Zone**: Set up weight benches, dumbbells, and resistance bands in this area.
- **Stretching/Mobility Zone**: Keep a mat and space for yoga, stretching, or mobility exercises.

This division will help optimize the flow of your workouts and make it easier to navigate through your home gym.

Ventilation and Lighting

Proper ventilation and lighting are essential for creating an inviting and comfortable home gym. If possible, position your gym in a spot with natural light. Natural light can boost your mood and energy levels during workouts. If natural light is limited, invest in good quality lighting fixtures that provide ample brightness for your exercises.

Ventilation is also crucial. Ensure there's good airflow to keep the space fresh and odor-free. If your gym area doesn't have windows, consider using fans or an air purifier to maintain air quality.

Utilizing Wall Space

Don't overlook the potential of wall space when optimizing your home gym's layout. Utilize walls for storage solutions like racks or shelves to keep your equipment organized and easily accessible. Wall-mounted storage can free up floor space and make your gym look tidy.

Another great idea is to hang mirrors on the walls. Mirrors can help you check your form during exercises and create a sense of spaciousness, making the room feel larger than it actually is.

Considering Safety and Accessibility

Safety should always be a priority when designing your home gym layout. Ensure there is enough clearance around the equipment to avoid accidents or injuries. Be mindful of the placement of heavy equipment like weight benches or power racks, ensuring they are positioned securely and won't tip over.

Additionally, keep emergency exits clear and accessible at all times. It's important to have a safe environment where you can focus on your workouts without worrying about potential hazards.

Summary

Optimizing the space and layout of your home gym is crucial for a successful workout experience. Start by measuring your space accurately and considering the flow of movement. Divide the space into functional zones, utilize wall space for storage and mirrors, and ensure proper ventilation and lighting. Prioritize safety and accessibility throughout the layout process. By taking these steps, you can create a well-organized and efficient home gym that motivates you to achieve your fitness goals.

So, let's get to work and create the perfect home gym setup that will keep you inspired and energized for every workout!

Chapter 5: Creating Effective Workout Routines

When it comes to achieving your fitness goals, having a well-structured and effective workout routine is essential. In this chapter, we'll explore the key elements of creating workout routines that are not only challenging but also sustainable and tailored to your specific needs. Let's dive in and discover how to design a fitness plan that works for you.

Understanding Your Fitness Goals

Before diving into the world of workout routines, it's crucial to have a clear understanding of your fitness goals. Are you looking to build strength, lose weight, increase endurance, or improve overall fitness? Defining your objectives will help guide your workout routine and ensure it aligns with what you want to achieve.

Consider Your Time Availability

Another factor to consider when creating your workout routine is your time availability. Determine how many days per week you can dedicate to exercising and the duration of each session. This information will assist in structuring your routine to make the most of the time you have available. For instance, if you can work out three times a week for

an hour each session, you'll plan differently than if
you have five days a week but only 30 minutes
each day.

Include All Components of Fitness

An effective workout routine should include
components that address all aspects of fitness:
cardiovascular exercise, strength training, flexibility,
and mobility. Incorporate exercises from each
category into your routine to ensure a well-rounded
approach to fitness.

Cardiovascular Exercise

Cardiovascular exercise, also known as aerobic
exercise, is essential for improving heart health and
stamina. It involves activities that elevate your heart
rate, such as running, cycling, swimming, or using
cardio equipment like treadmills or ellipticals.
Decide how many days per week you will dedicate
to cardio and choose activities you enjoy to make it
more sustainable. For example, you might plan to
do a 30-minute run on Mondays, a cycling session
on Wednesdays, and a swimming workout on
Fridays.

Strength Training

Strength training plays a vital role in building
muscle, improving bone density, and increasing
metabolism. Incorporate exercises that target major

muscle groups, such as squats, deadlifts, lunges, chest presses, and rows. Consider the equipment you have in your home gym, such as dumbbells, resistance bands, or weight machines, and design your routine accordingly. A sample strength training schedule might include upper body workouts on Tuesdays and Thursdays and lower body workouts on Saturdays.

Flexibility and Mobility

Flexibility and mobility exercises are often neglected but are crucial for maintaining joint health and preventing injuries. Include stretches and mobility exercises that target different areas of your body, such as yoga, Pilates, or dynamic warm-up routines. Devote at least a few minutes at the beginning and end of each workout to focus on flexibility and mobility. For instance, you could start each session with a five-minute dynamic warm-up and end with a ten-minute yoga flow.

Progressive Overload and Variation

To continue making progress and avoid hitting a plateau, it's essential to incorporate progressive overload and variation into your workout routine. Progressive overload means gradually increasing the intensity, duration, or repetitions of your exercises over time. Variation involves changing exercises, rep ranges, or workout formats to keep your body challenged and prevent boredom. For example, you might increase your squat weight by 5% every two weeks or swap out traditional push-ups for decline push-ups to increase difficulty.

Listen to Your Body

Lastly, always listen to your body and make adjustments to your routine when necessary. Pay attention to how your body responds to certain exercises and adjust the intensity or volume accordingly. Rest and recovery are equally important, so schedule rest days to allow your body to repair and regenerate. For instance, if you notice persistent soreness or fatigue, it might be time to incorporate an extra rest day or focus on lower-intensity activities like walking or gentle stretching.

Putting It All Together

Now that you have a comprehensive understanding of how to create an effective workout routine, let's put it all together. Here's a sample weekly workout plan:

- **Monday**: 30-minute run (cardio) + 10 minutes of yoga (flexibility)
- **Tuesday**: Upper body strength training (dumbbells) + 5-minute dynamic warm-up + 10-minute stretch
- **Wednesday**: 45-minute cycling (cardio) + 10 minutes of Pilates (mobility)

- **Thursday**: Lower body strength training (squats, lunges) + 5-minute dynamic warm-up + 10-minute stretch
- **Friday**: Swimming session (cardio) + 10 minutes of foam rolling (recovery)
- **Saturday**: Full-body strength training (combination of upper and lower body) + 10-minute yoga flow (flexibility)
- **Sunday**: Rest day or gentle walk + stretching

By considering your fitness goals, time availability, and incorporating all components of fitness, you can create an effective workout routine that keeps you motivated and on track toward achieving your desired results. Remember to constantly reassess and modify your routine as you progress along your fitness journey. With consistency and dedication, you'll be well on your way to achieving your best body.

Chapter 6: Incorporating Progressive Overload

Incorporating progressive overload into your home gym routine is essential for continuous growth and improvement. Progressive overload refers to gradually increasing the demands placed on your muscles to force them to adapt and become stronger over time. It's a fundamental principle of exercise that allows you to make consistent progress and avoid plateaus.

Understanding Progressive Overload

Progressive overload can be achieved in various ways, including:

1. Increasing Resistance: As your muscles become accustomed to a certain weight, you need to increase the resistance to continue challenging them. This can be done by adding more weight, using resistance bands, or choosing heavier dumbbells or barbells. For example, if you've been bench pressing 50 pounds, try increasing it to 55 pounds once you feel comfortable.

2. Increasing Repetitions: Another way to incorporate progressive overload is by increasing the number of repetitions you perform with a given weight. As you become stronger, you can gradually add more repetitions to each set, pushing your muscles to work harder. If you've been doing 8 reps of squats, try moving up to 10 or 12 reps.

3. Increasing Sets: Adding additional sets to your workout routine is another effective way to progressively overload your muscles. This increases the overall volume of work performed and places greater stress on your muscles. If you typically do 3 sets of bicep curls, try adding a fourth set.

4. Reducing Rest Periods: Shortening the rest periods between sets challenges your muscles to work harder and endure more stress. By reducing rest periods, you create a more intense workout environment that promotes muscle growth and adaptation. If you usually rest for 2 minutes between sets, try reducing it to 90 seconds.

5. Increasing Training Frequency: Training more frequently provides your muscles with more opportunities to adapt and grow. However, it's important to balance frequency with adequate rest and recovery to avoid overtraining. If you train each muscle group once a week, consider increasing it to twice a week.

Benefits of Progressive Overload

Incorporating progressive overload into your home gym routine offers several benefits, including:

1. Increased Strength: Progressive overload helps stimulate muscle fibers, leading to increased strength and muscle growth. By gradually increasing the demands placed on your muscles, you can progressively strengthen them over time.

2. Improved Endurance: Progressive overload challenges your muscles to sustain higher workloads, leading to improved endurance. Whether you're performing cardio exercises or strength training, continuously challenging yourself will enhance your overall stamina.

3. Enhanced Muscle Definition: By consistently incorporating progressive overload, you can promote muscle hypertrophy and achieve a more defined and sculpted physique. As your muscles adapt and grow, they become more visible and defined.

4. Preventing Plateaus: Plateaus occur when your muscles adapt to a certain level of stress and stop making progress. Incorporating progressive overload ensures that your muscles constantly face new challenges, preventing plateaus and allowing for continuous growth.

Tips for Incorporating Progressive Overload

To effectively incorporate progressive overload into your home gym routine, consider the following tips:

1. Track Your Progress: Keep a workout journal or use a fitness app to track your exercises, sets, reps, and weights. This will allow you to monitor your progress over time and make informed decisions about when and how to increase the demands on your muscles.

2. Gradual Increases: Avoid making sudden and drastic increases in weight or volume, as this can increase the risk of injury. Instead, aim for gradual and consistent progress to give your muscles time to adapt.

3. Periodization: Implementing a structured periodization program can help you systematically vary the intensity and volume of your workouts. This involves alternating periods of higher intensity and lower intensity to optimize muscle adaptation and minimize the risk of overtraining.

4. Listen to Your Body: Pay attention to your body's signals and adjust your training accordingly. If you experience excessive fatigue, lack of progress, or persistent muscle soreness, it may be a sign that you need to modify your training load or give yourself more rest and recovery.

Conclusion

Incorporating progressive overload into your home gym routine is pivotal for achieving long-term fitness goals. By gradually increasing the demands placed on your muscles and consistently challenging yourself, you can continue making progress and avoid reaching a plateau. Remember to track your progress, make gradual increases, and listen to your body to ensure safe and effective training. Embrace the principle of progressive overload, and watch your strength, endurance, and muscle definition improve over time.

Continue reading to discover how to design effective workout routines and optimize your home gym setup in the next chapter.

Chapter 7: Implementing Cardiovascular Training

Cardiovascular training, commonly known as cardio, is an essential component of a well-rounded fitness routine. This chapter will guide you through the importance of cardiovascular exercise and provide tips for implementing it effectively in your home gym setup.

The Benefits of Cardiovascular Training

Cardiovascular training offers numerous benefits for both physical and mental well-being. Incorporating regular cardio workouts into your routine can:

1. **Improve Heart Health:** Cardio exercises such as running, cycling, and swimming help strengthen the heart muscles and improve its efficiency. This, in turn, enhances blood circulation and reduces the risk of cardiovascular diseases.
2. **Enhance Endurance:** Regular cardio workouts gradually increase your aerobic capacity, allowing you to perform physical activities for longer periods without fatigue. This increased endurance can benefit other aspects of your fitness routine and daily life.
3. **Burn Calories and Aid Weight Loss:** Cardio exercises are excellent

calorie-burners. Engaging in activities like jogging, brisk walking, or HIIT (High-Intensity Interval Training) helps create a calorie deficit and supports weight loss goals.

4. **Boost Energy Levels:** Regular cardio workouts stimulate the release of endorphins, often referred to as "feel-good" hormones. These hormones help elevate your mood and energy levels, leaving you feeling refreshed and ready to tackle the day.

5. **Reduce Stress and Anxiety:** Cardiovascular exercises act as a natural stress reliever, reducing the levels of stress hormones such as cortisol and promoting a sense of relaxation and mental well-being.

Choosing the Right Cardiovascular Equipment

When setting up your home gym, selecting appropriate cardiovascular equipment that aligns with your fitness goals and space constraints is crucial. Here are some popular options to consider:

1. **Treadmills:** Treadmills are versatile cardio machines that allow you to walk, jog, or run in the comfort of your own home. Look for features such as speed control, incline settings, and safety features like emergency stop buttons.

2. **Ellipticals:** Ellipticals provide low-impact cardio workouts that engage both upper and lower body muscles. These machines are ideal for those who want a joint-friendly option that still provides an intense cardiovascular workout.

3. **Stationary Bikes:** Stationary bikes come in various forms, such as upright bikes, recumbent bikes, and indoor cycling bikes. They offer a convenient way to get a cardio workout while minimizing impact on your joints.

4. **Jump Ropes:** Jump ropes are affordable and portable cardio tools that allow you to engage in a high-intensity workout, improving your coordination and agility. They are an excellent choice for those with limited space or a tight budget.

5. **Mini Trampolines:** Mini trampolines, also known as rebounders, provide a fun and effective cardiovascular workout. They are low-impact and can be used for various exercises such as jogging, jumping jacks, or dance workouts.

Designing Cardiovascular Workouts

To make the most out of your cardiovascular training in your home gym, it's essential to design effective workout routines. Consider the following factors:

1. **Frequency:** Aim for at least 150 minutes of moderate-intensity cardio or 75 minutes of vigorous-intensity cardio per week. Distribute these sessions throughout the week based on your preference and schedule.
2. **Intensity:** Adjust the intensity of your cardio workouts based on your fitness level and goals. High-intensity interval training (HIIT) and steady-state cardio both have their benefits, so incorporate a mix of both into your routine.
3. **Variety:** Keep your cardio workouts interesting and prevent boredom by trying different activities. Alternate between using different equipment, exploring outdoor options like running or cycling, or incorporating dance cardio or aerobic classes into your routine.
4. **Warm-up and Cool-down:** Prioritize a proper warm-up and cool-down period before and after your cardio sessions. This helps prepare your body for the workout, prevents injuries, and aids in recovery.
5. **Progression:** Gradually increase the duration, intensity, or resistance of your cardio workouts to challenge your body and continually improve your cardiovascular fitness. This progression ensures that you keep pushing your limits and avoid plateaus.

Sample Cardiovascular Workout Plan

Here's a sample plan to help you get started:

1. **Warm-up:** Start with 5-10 minutes of light cardio, such as walking or gentle jogging, to get your heart rate up and muscles warmed.
2. **Workout:**
    - **Day 1: Treadmill Intervals**
        - 5 minutes warm-up walk
        - 1 minute sprint, 2 minutes walk (repeat 6 times)
        - 5 minutes cool-down walk
    - **Day 2: Elliptical Workout**
        - 5 minutes easy pace
        - 3 minutes moderate pace, 1 minute high resistance (repeat 5 times)
        - 5 minutes easy pace cool-down
    - **Day 3: Rest or Light Activity**
        - Gentle yoga or a leisurely walk
    - **Day 4: Stationary Bike HIIT**
        - 5 minutes warm-up
        - 30 seconds sprint, 1 minute easy pace (repeat 10 times)
        - 5 minutes cool-down
    - **Day 5: Jump Rope Circuit**
        - 5 minutes warm-up
        - 1 minute jump rope, 1 minute rest (repeat 10 times)

- 5 minutes cool-down
  - **Day 6: Outdoor Run or Cycle**
    - Choose a scenic route for a moderate 30-45 minute session
  - **Day 7: Active Recovery**
    - Light stretching or a slow-paced walk

Conclusion

Implementing cardiovascular training in your home gym setup adds a dynamic and vital component to your overall fitness routine. Whether you choose equipment like treadmills or opt for more budget-friendly options like jump ropes, consistency is key. Regular cardio workouts will help you reap the numerous benefits associated with improved heart health, increased endurance, weight management, stress reduction, and overall well-being. So get ready to lace up your sneakers and embrace the cardio journey in the comfort of your home gym.

In the next chapter, we will explore the importance of flexibility and mobility training and how to incorporate them into your fitness routine for comprehensive health benefits.

Chapter 8: Focusing on Flexibility and Mobility

Flexibility and mobility are crucial components of overall fitness and play a significant role in preventing injuries, improving posture, and enhancing athletic performance. In this chapter, we will explore the importance of flexibility and mobility exercises and how to effectively incorporate them into your home gym routine.

The Importance of Flexibility and Mobility

Flexibility refers to the range of motion around a joint, while mobility refers to the ability to move a joint freely through its full range of motion. Both flexibility and mobility are important for maintaining good posture, proper movement patterns, and joint health. Regular flexibility and mobility exercises can help:

- Improve muscle and joint elasticity
- Enhance athletic performance and prevent injuries
- Alleviate muscle tightness and reduce muscle soreness
- Promote better blood circulation and nutrient delivery to muscles
- Correct imbalances and improve posture
- Enhance overall movement quality

Incorporating Flexibility and Mobility Exercises

To effectively incorporate flexibility and mobility exercises into your home gym routine, consider the following tips:

Dynamic Warm-Up

Before starting your workout, it's essential to warm up your muscles and prepare them for physical activity. A dynamic warm-up routine that includes dynamic stretching exercises can help improve flexibility and mobility. Dynamic stretches involve controlled movements that gently take your body through a range of motion. Some examples of dynamic stretches include:

- **Arm Circles:** Gently rotate your arms in large circles to warm up your shoulder joints.
- **Leg Swings:** Swing your legs forward and backward, and side to side, to warm up your hip joints.
- **Walking Lunges:** Step forward into a lunge position, alternating legs as you move.
- **Hip Circles:** Rotate your hips in a circular motion to loosen up your hip joints.

Static Stretching

After your workout or as a standalone session, dedicate time to perform static stretching exercises. Static stretches are held for a period of time, usually around 30 seconds, and target specific muscles or muscle groups. Some common static stretches include:

- **Hamstring Stretches:** Sit on the floor with one leg extended and the other bent. Reach toward your toes on the extended leg.
- **Calf Stretches:** Stand facing a wall with one foot forward and the other back. Press your back heel into the ground.
- **Quadriceps Stretches:** Stand on one leg and pull your other foot towards your buttocks.
- **Chest Stretches:** Clasp your hands behind your back and lift them slightly to open your chest.
- **Shoulder Stretches:** Bring one arm across your chest and use the other arm to hold it in place.

Remember to breathe deeply and relax into each stretch, avoiding any bouncing or jerking movements.

Yoga and Pilates

Yoga and Pilates are excellent practices to improve flexibility and mobility. These disciplines incorporate a wide range of movements and positions, targeting both major muscle groups and smaller stabilizing muscles. Consider incorporating yoga or Pilates sessions into your home gym routine through online classes or instructional videos. These practices can enhance your flexibility, mobility, strength, and overall mind-body connection.

Foam Rolling and Self-Myofascial Release

Foam rolling and self-myofascial release techniques involve using foam rollers, massage balls, or other tools to apply pressure to certain areas of your body. This helps release muscle tension, improve circulation, and enhance flexibility. By incorporating foam rolling and self-myofascial release into your home gym routine, you can target specific muscle groups, such as your calves, quads, hamstrings, and back. Spend a few minutes rolling over each area, focusing on any tight or tender spots.

Stretching Accessories

Consider investing in stretching accessories to enhance your flexibility and mobility routine. These accessories may include:

- **Resistance Bands:** These can be used to assist with stretching and increase the difficulty of certain exercises.

- **Yoga Blocks:** Provide support and help maintain proper alignment during stretches.
- **Stability Balls:** Useful for improving balance and core strength while stretching.
- **Stretching Straps:** Assist in deepening stretches or reaching difficult positions.

Conclusion

Flexibility and mobility should be prioritized in any well-rounded home gym routine. Incorporating dynamic warm-ups, static stretching exercises, yoga or Pilates sessions, foam rolling, and utilizing stretching accessories can improve your overall flexibility, mobility, and movement quality. Remember to listen to your body, progress at your own pace, and always prioritize proper form to avoid injury.

By integrating these practices, you'll enhance your physical performance, reduce the risk of injury, and enjoy a more balanced and effective fitness routine.

Chapter 9: Establishing a Routine and Consistency

Hey there! Let's talk about one of the most important aspects of achieving your fitness goals: establishing a routine and maintaining consistency. Whether you're just starting out or you've been working out for a while, having a structured plan and sticking to it can make all the difference in your journey to a healthier lifestyle. So, let's dive into how you can create a routine that works for you and helps you stay on track.

The Importance of a Routine

Having a routine provides structure and discipline, which are essential for long-term success. When you have a set schedule for your workouts, it becomes easier to prioritize exercise and make it a non-negotiable part of your day. Plus, a routine helps create a habit, making it easier to stay consistent and motivated.

Understanding Your Fitness Goals

Before you establish your exercise routine, it's important to clearly define your fitness goals. Are you looking to lose weight, build muscle, increase endurance, or improve flexibility? Understanding your goals will help you determine the types of workouts and exercises that are most effective in achieving them.

Considering Your Time Availability

When creating your routine, consider how much time you can realistically dedicate to your workouts each day. Take into account your work schedule, family commitments, and other responsibilities. It's better to have a shorter, more intense workout that you can consistently stick to than a longer workout that you struggle to fit into your schedule.

Including All Components of Fitness

A well-rounded exercise routine should include all components of fitness: cardiovascular exercise, strength training, flexibility, and mobility. Each component plays a vital role in achieving optimal health and fitness.

Cardiovascular Exercise

Cardiovascular exercise, also known as cardio, is important for improving heart health, boosting endurance, and burning calories. Incorporate activities like running, cycling, swimming, or using cardio machines into your routine. Aim for at least 150 minutes of moderate-intensity cardio exercise per week.

Strength Training

Strength training helps build muscle, increase metabolism, and improve overall strength and stability. Include exercises that target all major muscle groups, such as squats, lunges, deadlifts, push-ups, and pull-ups. Aim for at least two to three strength training sessions per week.

Flexibility and Mobility

Flexibility and mobility exercises are essential for maintaining joint health, preventing injuries, and improving overall flexibility. Incorporate static and dynamic stretching, as well as exercises that focus on mobility and range of motion, such as yoga or Pilates. Aim to stretch and perform mobility exercises at least two to three times per week.

Listening to Your Body and Making Adjustments

While consistency is important, it's equally crucial to listen to your body and make adjustments when needed. There will be days when you feel tired or sore, and it's okay to take a break or modify your workout. It's also important to challenge yourself by increasing the intensity or difficulty of your workouts as your fitness level improves.

The Importance of Rest and Recovery

Rest and recovery are vital components of any exercise routine. Your body needs time to repair and rebuild muscle tissue after intense workouts. Make sure to incorporate rest days into your routine to allow your body to recover and reduce the risk of overtraining and burnout.

Creating a Consistent Routine

To establish a consistent routine, consider the following tips:

- **Set a Specific Time for Your Workouts**: Pick a time that works best for you and stick to it. Whether it's first thing in the morning, during lunch, or in the evening, make it a part of your daily schedule.
- **Choose Activities and Exercises You Enjoy**: If you enjoy your workouts, you're more likely to stick with them. Find exercises that you look forward to doing.
- **Break Your Routine into Manageable Chunks**: Focus on different muscle groups on different days or divide your cardio and strength training sessions. This can help keep your workouts varied and interesting.
- **Utilize Technology Tools**: Use fitness apps or workout journals to track your progress and hold yourself accountable. Seeing your progress can be a great motivator.
- **Surround Yourself with a Supportive Environment**: Join a fitness community, find a workout buddy, or connect with

like-minded individuals. Having support can make a big difference in staying motivated.

In Conclusion

Establishing a routine and maintaining consistency are key to achieving your fitness goals. By understanding your goals, considering your time availability, including all components of fitness, listening to your body, and prioritizing rest and recovery, you can create a routine that works for you and sets you up for long-term success in your home gym.

So, let's get organized, stay consistent, and watch those fitness goals become a reality!

Chapter 10: Evolving Your Home Gym Setup

As you continue on your fitness journey, it's important to recognize that your home gym setup is not set in stone. Just as your fitness goals may evolve over time, so too should your gym environment. In this final chapter, we will explore the concept of evolving your home gym setup to ensure that it continues to meet your changing needs and preferences.

Assessing Your Progress

Before making any changes to your home gym, it's crucial to assess your progress and evaluate whether your current setup is still effective in helping you achieve your fitness goals. Take some time to reflect on your workouts, track your progress, and consider any areas for improvement. This self-reflection will provide valuable insights into what changes might be necessary to keep pushing yourself forward. Are you hitting your goals, or do you feel stuck? Is there any equipment you rarely use? Are there new types of workouts you're interested in trying? Answering these questions can help guide your decisions.

Expanding Your Equipment

As you become more experienced and your fitness level improves, you may find that your current equipment no longer challenges you enough. This is an excellent opportunity to invest in new and more advanced equipment that will allow you to continue progressing in your fitness journey. Consider adding items such as resistance bands with higher tension, heavier weights, or even specialized equipment for specific types of training, such as agility cones or battle ropes.

Tips for Expanding Your Equipment:

1. **Identify Gaps**: Look at your current workouts and identify areas where you feel limited. Maybe your dumbbells are too light, or you lack equipment for cardio workouts.
2. **Set Priorities**: Decide which new equipment will have the most significant impact on your workouts. Prioritize these items based on your budget and space.
3. **Research and Invest**: Take the time to research the best options within your budget. Investing in high-quality equipment can provide better performance and longevity.

Introducing New Training Modalities

Keeping your workouts fresh and engaging is key to staying motivated and preventing boredom. Explore new training modalities and techniques that you haven't tried before. This could include incorporating bodyweight exercises, HIIT (High-Intensity Interval Training) workouts, TRX suspension training, or even virtual fitness classes. By introducing variety to your workouts, you'll challenge your body in new ways and continue to see progress.

Ideas for New Training Modalities:

- **Bodyweight Exercises**: Push-ups, pull-ups, and squats can be incredibly effective without any equipment.
- **HIIT Workouts**: These high-intensity routines can be done with minimal equipment and are great for burning fat and improving cardiovascular health.
- **TRX Suspension Training**: This versatile equipment uses your body weight and gravity to provide a challenging workout.
- **Virtual Fitness Classes**: Platforms like Peloton, Beachbody, or YouTube offer a wide range of classes that can add variety and excitement to your routine.

Reorganizing and Optimizing Space

As you accumulate more equipment and explore new training modalities, you may need to reorganize and optimize your space to accommodate these changes. Consider rearranging your layout to create separate zones for cardio, strength training, and stretching. Explore creative storage solutions to keep your equipment organized and easily accessible. Additionally, ensure that your gym space remains safe and clutter-free by periodically reviewing and updating your layout.

Steps to Optimize Your Space:

1. **Create Zones**: Designate specific areas for different types of workouts, such as a cardio corner, a strength training section, and a stretching area.
2. **Use Vertical Space**: Install shelves or wall-mounted racks to store equipment like dumbbells, kettlebells, and resistance bands.
3. **Keep It Clean**: Regularly tidy up and reorganize your gym space to keep it inviting and functional.

Adding Motivational Elements

Sometimes, all it takes is a little motivation to keep you on track and excited about your workouts.

Consider adding motivational elements to your home gym setup, such as inspirational quotes, posters of your fitness idols, or a dedicated space for a vision board where you can display your fitness goals. These visual reminders will help keep you focused and committed to your fitness journey.

Ideas for Motivational Elements:

- **Inspirational Quotes**: Frame your favorite quotes and hang them where you can see them during your workouts.
- **Vision Board**: Create a board with images and notes that represent your fitness goals and dreams.
- **Music and Media**: Set up a sound system or TV to play your favorite workout tunes or fitness videos.

Seeking Professional Guidance

As you progress in your fitness journey, you may reach a point where you desire professional guidance to take your workouts to the next level. Consider hiring a personal trainer or fitness coach who can provide personalized programming, technique correction, and ongoing support. They can help you optimize your home gym setup and tailor your workouts according to your specific goals and abilities.

Benefits of Professional Guidance:

- **Personalized Workouts**: Get routines tailored to your goals and fitness level.
- **Expert Advice**: Learn proper form and techniques to prevent injuries.
- **Accountability**: Stay motivated and on track with regular check-ins and progress assessments.

Conclusion

Your home gym setup should be a dynamic and ever-evolving space that grows with you as you progress in your fitness journey. By regularly assessing your progress, expanding your equipment, exploring new training modalities, optimizing your space, adding motivational elements, and seeking professional guidance when needed, you can ensure that your home gym remains a place of inspiration, growth, and success. Remember, the key is to always be open to change and adapt your setup as your needs and goals evolve.

Your fitness journey is unique, and so should be your home gym. Embrace the process, stay committed, and enjoy the incredible benefits of working out in a space designed just for you. Happy training!